With Much Love
To Jeff, Laura & Baby Boy Schmerin
   June 2, 2011

By Grandparents Mary Los & Charlie Schmerin

In honor of the announcement of
the announcement
the arrival of Baby Schmerin 4-2-11

The Miracle Within

JACK McCUBBIN, M.D.

with Cathy Schaffer

Barkman Creek Press

Barkman Creek Press
www.barkmancreekpress.com
www.themiraclewithin.com

ISBN-10: 0-9786336-0-1
ISBN-13: 978-0-9786336-0-8

Photos are 2006 copyrighted material of Photoresearchers Inc.,
Phototake USA , and Siemens Medical Solutions.

Cover photos: 2006 copyrighted material of Photoresearchers Inc, and Painet Photos.

Cover design: George Foster, www.fostercovers.com
Interior design: Liz Tufte, www.folio-bookworks.com

Printed in Canada

DEDICATION

Liza Boyd McCubbin is a loving mother and wife whose contribution to this project — and all others — is invaluable. Without her support and patience this book would not have been possible. It is because of her love that I am able to present this work as a *labor of love* to all women who are and will be mothers. I dedicate this to *all of you and the Miracle Within You.*

— Jack

Denise, Rachal and Danny — may you recognize what a gift life is and the tremendous gift you are to me. To my husband Bear, you are the love of my life.

To my Lord in Heaven, the great Creator, the writer of all great books, thank you for these words. Without you, there is no life.

— Cathy

CONTENTS

INTRODUCTION

"Some people call it butterfly wings, or champagne bubbles,
or mermaids blowing kisses. I call it a miracle."
—Betty Williamson

When you look into the mirror what do you see? Do you notice the color of your skin, the shape of your nose or the beauty of your smile? Do people tell you that you look like your mother or your father? Do you ever stop and wonder how you began? Did you know that the way you look now was determined the exact moment when sperm and egg united? Did you know that the makeup and personality of the baby you are now carrying was determined many years ago when you and the baby's father were still in the womb?

Pregnancy is a creative work in progress. Your unborn baby represents the most complex litany of systems management ever imagined. When sperm and egg meet, life begins to unfold in a series of cell divisions and development that have only recently been witnessed. In the past we have been limited to viewing the miracle only from the outside of the human body. Today, in this book, we can give you a glimpse of your pregnancy and its progression from the inside. We will show you what miracles actually look like.

This book is not intended to be all inclusive. Use it along with other resources such as the internet, additional books and your healthcare provider to inform you about your pregnancy.

The book is divided into trimesters that celebrate and acknowledge the unique changes that are occurring. As you progress through your pregnancy it is our hope that this book will help you to envision "The Miracle Within."

IN THE BEGINNING. . .

"Motherhood: All love begins and ends there."
~Robert Browning

This is a microscopic photo of an egg being released from the ovary.
With a gentle push, the egg is released to be tenderly caught by the fallopian tube
and then it's off to discover its destiny.

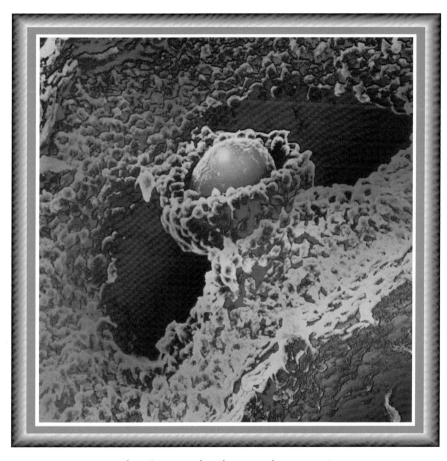

Photo: ©P. Bagavandoss/Photo Researchers, Inc. 2006

"If I had my life
to live over,
instead of wishing away
nine months of pregnancy,
I'd have cherished
every moment and realized
that the wonderment
growing inside me
was the only chance in life
to assist God in a miracle."

— Erma Bombeck

Y̲ou may not recognize the marvel that has just occurred within you.

According to experts in the areas of fertilization and conception, getting pregnant isn't as easy as it may seem. In fact, your chances of getting pregnant are only about twenty-five percent each cycle. It takes most couples who are *trying* to get pregnant six to twelve months before they conceive.

OVULATION

Let's start at the beginning, before you were even born. Your ovaries had millions of eggs while you were in the womb. By puberty your eggs had decreased to around 200,000 – 400,000. Every month, beginning in puberty, a single egg is selected for final growth and release. In preparation for a fertilized egg, the uterus grows a thick lining. When there is no fertilized egg the uterus sheds this lining and your monthly cycle begins. The first day of bleeding is day one of your cycle.

When an ovary releases an egg it's called ovulation. Ovulation begins approximately two weeks from the first day of bleeding. Its release is not an explosive event (although it may feel that way at times) but rather a gentle one, followed by a tender rescue by the fallopian tube. When an egg is released it represents the largest cell in a woman's body. It is barely visible to the naked eye and would be about the size of a pencil dot.

"It's the state of being pregnant, as if you're weaving a house for your child out of your own body, and it takes all your energy, all your attention."

– Hilma Wolitzer
American Writer

Out of the thousands of sperm released,
only one, the "hero sperm," unites with the nucleus of the egg.
When sperm come into the vicinity of an egg,
their tail movement becomes more forceful and erratic,
propelling them towards their target.
This forceful tail motion helps the sperm to penetrate the egg.

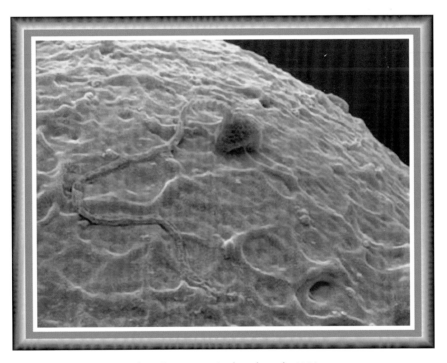

Photo: ©Mona Lisa/Eurelios/Phototake 2006

The egg that is selected for release is surrounded by fluid and specialized protective cells. While inside the fallopian tube, the egg floats in fluid, propelled by the delicate movement of hair-like projections (cilia) toward the uterus. The egg has only 12 to 24 hours to live if it is not fertilized. After that time, it will die if union with a sperm has not taken place. On the other hand, sperm will live for days and have been found still mobile even several days following sexual intercourse.

"... for when a child is born the mother also is born again."

– Gilbert Parker "Parables of a Province"

At the time of ejaculation during intercourse, the tiny sperm must travel approximately 7 inches from the site in the vagina where they were deposited, to the site of fertilization in the upper one-third of the uterine tube. This journey usually takes about two hours.

Contractions within the uterus and tubes enable the microscopic sperm to travel this distance rapidly. Dead sperm can travel as rapidly as live ones once inside the uterus!

Hundreds of sperm may actually reach the upper end of the tube. Do these extra sperm benefit in fertilization? Probably so. It is thought that "helper" sperm utilize enzymes that break down a protective layer around the egg so that the "hero sperm" can unite with the nucleus of the egg.

When you think about all the things that had to happen before you could conceive, you might consider yourself very special. You have been given a gift. Inside your body sperm and egg have met and become one.

FERTLIZATION

At the moment of fertilization, the nuclei of the sperm and the egg fuse, and the new being formed is called a *zygote*. The cells begin to multiply rapidly, growing at an unprecedented rate. The zygote continues to move through your fallopian tube towards the uterus, its new home for the next nine months. All of this is occurring as you sleep, get up in the morning and get ready for work and go about your daily routine.

Each day this tiny little sac of cells is changing and growing. At this point you probably aren't even aware of the wonderful changes occurring within you. You haven't even yet missed a period. The process of rapid cell division into many cells is called *cleavage*. The one cell zygote is "cleaved" into hundreds of cells. The first cell division occurs about thirty hours after fertilization. Each division makes smaller cells. Although many more cells result, the overall mass remains unchanged. Certain of the cells which are cleaved are destined to become the baby itself, while others are destined to become placenta and membranes.

On the third day after fertilization, this new entity is near the junction of the fallopian tube and uterus and has assumed the shape of a small, hollow ball about the size of a pinhead. It now enters into the uterus and will spend another three days floating there.

"It is not until you become a mother that your judgment slowly turns to compassion and understanding."

–Erma Bombeck
(1927-1996)
American Writer

Within 24 hours after fertilization, the fertilized egg divides in half,
creating two parts. The new entity formed is called a zygote.
The cells begin to multiply rapidly, growing at an unprecedented rate.
It splits from two to four, four to eight, and so on,
getting tighter and tighter until the cells are almost fused together.

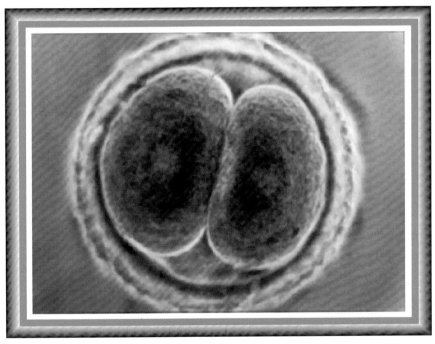

Photo: ©ICAM/Mona Lisa/Eurelios/Phototake 2006

This is your fertilized egg moving down your fallopian tube.
Small little finger-like projections called cilia move the egg forward.
On the third or fourth day after conception, the fertilized egg has divided
sixteen times and will reach the junction of the fallopian tube and the uterus.

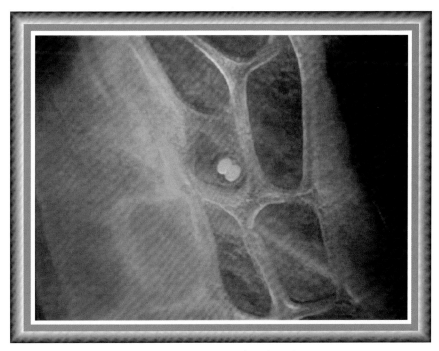

Photo: ©ICAM/Mona Lisa/Eurelios/Phototake 2006

On the fifth or sixth day,
the zygote settles down into its new home
and begins the process known as implantation.
This is a fertilized egg with a zona pellucida (egg coat).
The egg sheds this protected layer after arriving
in the womb and implanting in to the uterine wall.

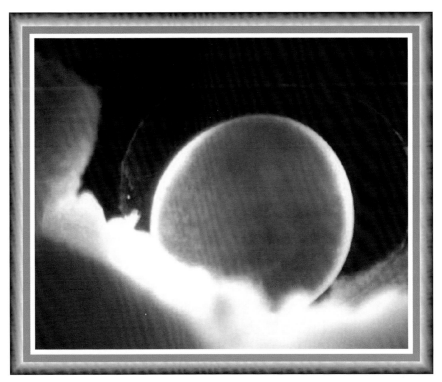

Photo: ©ICAM/Mona Lisa/Eurelios/Phototake 2006

On the fifth or sixth day, the zygote settles down into its new home and begins the process known as implantation. Most times implantation occurs high in the uterus and more commonly on its back wall, rather than the front one.

BOY OR GIRL?

Sperm and egg each carry half the number of genes that the baby will possess. Try to picture the microscopic miracle that is going on inside of you. Imagine the dividing cells are the ones that will give your baby your blue eyes or the father's dark hair. Envision your baby with grandmother's beautiful smile or grandfather's great personality. Because both of you have contributed 23 chromosomes to the developing zygote the possibilities are endless.

The BIG question is whether it will be a boy or a girl. That is determined by the father. The mother always carries XX chromosomes which are the female chromosomes. The father carries the XY chromosomes. If he contributes an X chromosome the baby will be a girl (XX). If he contributes the Y chromosome the baby will be a boy (XY). This is the only time during the pregnancy the baby relies on the father to influence the outcome. The rest of the pregnancy will depend entirely on the woman and her body for the development of the new life!

"When God thought of mother, He must have laughed with satisfaction, and framed it quickly – so rich, so deep, so divine, so full of soul, power, and beauty, was the conception."

–Henry Ward Beecher

THE FIRST TRIMESTER

"You are the caretaker of the generations, you are the birth giver,"
the sun told the woman. "You will be the carrier of this universe."
—Brule Sioux Sun Creation Myth

By the time you take your pregnancy test,
your little zygote has become an embryo
and has undergone quite a few changes.
The "bag of waters" forms
from this network of cells
as well as the yolk sac
(see the tiny group of cells on the right)
which will provide nourishment
for your embryo during its early development.

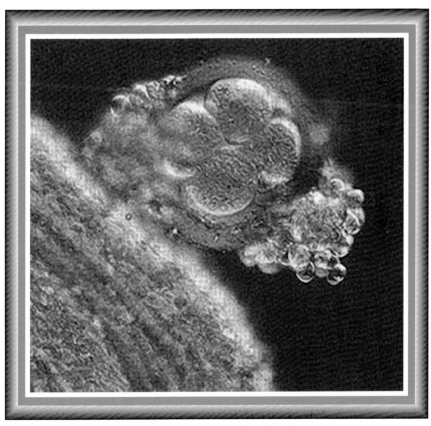

Photo: ©ICAM/Mona Lisa/Eurelios/Phototake 2006

ARE YOU OR AREN'T YOU?

Although you have not missed a period, you may be feeling like you have the flu. Perhaps you got up this morning and felt nauseous. Maybe you are noticing that your breasts are slightly tender or you are just dragging these last few days. You hear this little whisper within that suggests you might be pregnant, but you don't pay too much attention to it. But you decide to try one of those over the counter pregnancy tests just to put your mind at rest. This test measures hCG (*human Chorionic Gonadotropin*), a hormone secreted by the developing placenta shortly after the egg implants itself into the uterus. hCG is measured in thousandths of International Units or mIU. In order to determine the sensitivity of a urine pregnancy test look for a lower mIU. For example a test that detects 20 mIU is more sensitive than a test that measures 50 mIU. Greater sensitivity equates earlier detection; a urine pregnancy test that detects 20 mIU's can detect a pregnancy 8 days after implantation. If you want even earlier detection a *blood* pregnancy test can detect hCG as low as 5 mIUs! This time, *your* test is positive.

"Her children arise up and call her blessed."

– Proverbs 31:28

FROM ZYGOTE TO EMBRYO

By the time you take your pregnancy test, your little zygote is now an embryo and has undergone quite a few changes. It has gone from a hollow ball of cells to a flat disc consisting of two layers. The "bag of waters" forms from this as well as the yolk sac that will provide nourishment for your embryo during its early development. There is a dramatic increase in size as the embryo develops three layers called the *ectoderm, endoderm*, and the *mesoderm*. Each of these layers will develop different systems. For example the *ectoderm* will form the skin, hair, nails, breasts, lens of the eyes, and enamel of the teeth. *Endodermal* structures are: lungs, liver, pancreas, bladder, thyroid gland, and lining of the intestines. The *mesodermal* layer includes the entire skeleton (except the skull), muscles, lymph system, spleen, the testes and ovaries.

> "Only mothers can think of the future — because they give birth to it in their children."
>
> – Maxim Gorky

During the next couple of weeks, as you tell your partner, family and friends the great news, your baby continues to astound. He/She changes from a three-layered disc to a cylinder with a head fold and a tail fold and is about the size of a lower case c. The earliest beginnings of an eye and ear are visible. A very primitive heart will begin to beat sometime around the fifth or sixth week. Blood cells and blood vessels are formed; but blood type was genetically determined at the moment of fertilization. A tube now represents the embryos central nervous system. The front part of this tube closes to create a primitive brain very early on.

Formation of neural tube (spinal cord) segments in an embryo.
Cells along the segments become the digestive tract, nerves,
and adrenal glands as well as other organs.
Also, blocks of tissue, called somites, begin to form pairs.
Eventually there will be more than 40 pairs.
Much of muscle, ligaments, cartilage,
and some bone and skin come from somites.

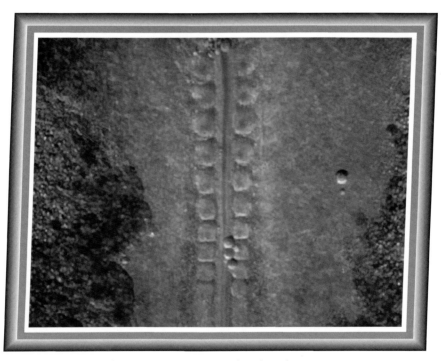

Photo: ©ICAM/Mona Lisa/Eurelios/Phototake 2006

GETTING THE WHITECOAT TREATMENT

Today you are going to see your healthcare provider because of your positive pregnancy test. He/She will examine you, probably do another pregnancy test, run some lab work and do a very thorough medical history. They may also order an ultrasound. By using an ultrasound your healthcare provider can detect your developing embryo. Ultrasound is a process that utilizes reflected sound waves (much like a submarine's sonar) to create a picture of internal body organs. In fact, ultrasound has become so sophisticated that your baby can be seen in 3D. The pictures are really amazing. Your healthcare provider may suggest doing a transvaginal ultrasound to examine your early pregnancy.

> "The heart of a mother is a deep abyss at the bottom of which you will always discover forgiveness."
>
> – Honoré de Balzac (1799 – 1850) French Writer

By placing the ultrasound probe inside the vagina, it is easier to see this tiny little being. A transvaginal ultrasound early in pregnancy can verify your pregnancy, ensure that it is within the uterus, detect multiple pregnancies, and make sure your tubes and ovaries appear normal. Typically, you will have a transvaginal ultrasound only in the very early stages of your pregnancy. Later ultrasounds will be done by moving a probe over your abdomen.

While you are at the doctor's office you tell him you have been feeling horrible. Nausea, breast tenderness, fatigue and increased frequency of urination have been contributing to some sleepless nights and some very rough mornings. Of course these are very common symptoms for most women at this period in a pregnancy. They are a consequence of the abundance of hormones produced by the placenta. You will start to feel better once this surge of hormones passes. In the meantime, it would be wise to have crackers, flat soda, water, gum and any other anti-nausea remedies near the bedside and in your desk at work. As for the fatigue, get family members to pitch in and help you. You should rest whenever you have an opportunity. Now is not the time to be superwoman.

Congratulate yourself. You have started prenatal care very early which is critical for your health as well as your unborn child's.

THE EARLY EMBRYO

By the time you are two weeks overdue for your period your little embryo is tube-shaped and about the same size as an uppercase "C". Its head fold is now very distinct from its tail fold. The embryo has a pointed tail and gill-like structures from which several other structures will develop, such as the lower jaw and voice box. There is a mouth opening, the beginning of an inner ear and a leg bud appears.

A simple one-chamber heart has formed and is beating. A partition forms in the heart from which the chambers of the heart will develop. The tube that represents the central nervous system now has three bubbles that will eventually form the brain. Nerves are beginning to form. Other

"Youth fades; love droops; the leaves of friendship fall; A mother's secret hope outlives them all."

– Oliver Wendell Holmes Jr.

organs are also present in very primitive form: lungs, liver, pancreas and thyroid.

Cells which will become sperm or eggs may be seen in the yolk sac wall.

These cells start migrating toward the site of the developing testes

or ovaries. They actually move with little feet-like projections

called pseudopods! The "germ" cells (future sperm or eggs) will

reach the ridge that represents the developing ovary or testes.

Once the cells have migrated, the yolk sac will begin to break

away and eventually disappear.

Your baby's heartbeat can be detected by ultrasound now.

The heart beats between 40 – 80 times per minute and it will

double in size this week. It is so large that it actually "bulges"

forward – not unlike a pregnant tummy.

"There is a religion in all deep love, but the love of a mother is the veil of a softer light between the heart and the heavenly Father."

– Samuel
Taylor Coleridge

6 TO 8 WEEKS

By the time you are four weeks overdue for your period your baby's head is very large in comparison to the rest its body. He/She no longer looks like a "C" and the trunk of the embryo appears longer. Your baby's upper lip is forming and the nose appears to have a tip. The eyes are positioned very far apart (about 160 degrees) so they appear to be on the sides of the head. Don't worry, they will move into the right position. Eyelids are beginning to form. The heart has achieved its final form and the intestine is so long now that it pushes (*herniates*) into the umbilical cord. While the intestine is in the cord, the appendix appears.

During this time, your embryo remains hard at work actively forming its organ systems. Around the seventh or eighth week your unborn baby measures about 0.3 of an inch. Hands and feet are recognizable and shaped like paddles. Arm buds are now larger than leg buds and there is an obvious tail. The backbone is now formed and the embryo's skin is so thin that it is actually transparent. A face is beginning to appear and some pigment can be detected in the iris of the eye.

Pretty soon your embryo begins to have reflexes! If its face is touched, the opposite side of its body will flex. Despite these spontaneous movements, most mothers will not feel any movement until somewhere between 16 and 20 weeks.

As the weeks after conception continue, the head is still relatively larger than the remainder of the body. Eyelids will begin to cover the eyes and the jaws are completely formed. External ears and a nose tip become distinguishable. If the baby is male, its testes are identifiable and the female system begins to disappear. Male cells appear which will make the testosterone hormone.

As the embryo continues to develop, the back of the embryo becomes less curved and a neck forms while the tail disappears. Its arms and legs are much longer and its elbow region appears. Most muscles throughout the body are attaining their final form.

"Mama was my greatest teacher, a teacher of compassion, love and fearlessness. If love is sweet as a flower, then my mother is that sweet flower of love."

– Stevie Wonder

By six weeks the baby is floating in amniotic fluid.
The little leg and arm buds are growing, and the lungs are developing.
The lenses of the eye form and the nostrils appear.

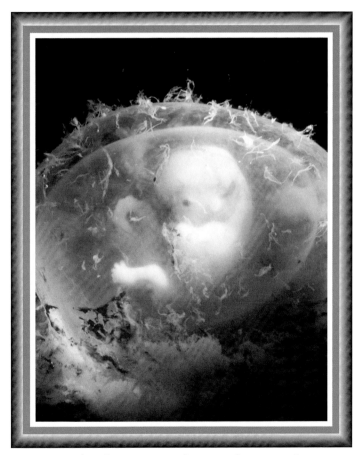

Photo: ©Dr G. Moscoso / Photo Researchers, Inc. 2006

By the time you are two weeks overdue for your period your little embryo
is tube-shaped and about the same size as an uppercase "C".
Its head fold is now very distinct from its tail fold.
The embryo has a pointed tail and gill-like structures
from which several other structures will develop,
such as the lower jaw and voice box.
There is a mouth opening and the beginning of an inner ear.

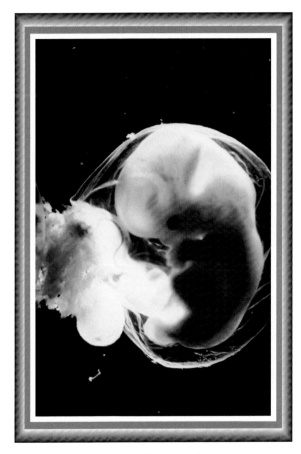

Photo: ©Petit Format / Photo Researchers, Inc. 2006.

At five or six weeks,
hands and feet are recognizable
and shaped like paddles.

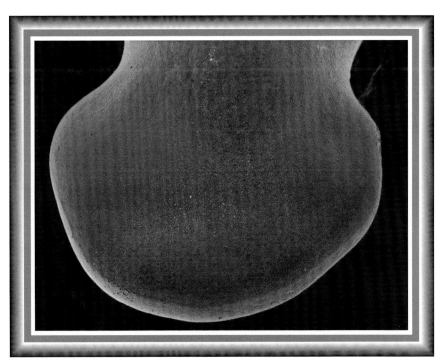

Photo: ©SPL / Photo Researchers, Inc. 2006

Beginning somewhere in the 8th week and until delivery, your unborn child will now be called a fetus and the adjective "fetal" is used to describe its structures and organs, for example, "fetal heart." Your baby has taken a huge leap forward!

DINING FOR TWO

Now is the time to consider making changes to your diet if you are someone who typically lives on fast-foods and junk. This type of eating will not sustain you or your growing baby for very long. It also causes you increased discomfort in the way of heartburn, nausea, vomiting and constipation.

So what is a healthy diet for a pregnant woman? Lots of research has been done in this area. Remember, *you* are the only source of nutrients for your baby. To begin with, you must provide the appropriate number of calories necessary. An adult woman usually needs about 1800 to 2200 calories per day depending on her activity level. With the addition of a growing fetus you will need to increase your calories by approximately 300 – 600 more calories a day. But don't get too excited, those extra calories can easily be met with a glass of milk and a sandwich.

What types of food should you eat during your pregnancy? You will find that rich foods such as cakes, cookies, heavy pasta, sauces and the like will give you incredible heartburn and for the most part, they are wasted

"I remember my mother's prayers, and they have always followed me. They have clung to me all my life."

– Abraham Lincoln
1809 – 1865

calories. Look for foods that are protein-rich and low in saturated fats such as fish, turkey, lean beef and chicken (skinless of course). You will need an extra thirty grams of protein every day. Proteins are used as building blocks for your baby's development.

Calcium is an extremely important part of your diet. Milk, low fat cheese, yogurt can all contribute calcium to your diet. Try to maintain your calcium intake around 1200 mg per day. A recent study from the faculty of nursing at Calgary University published in the Canadian Medical Association Journal in April 2006 showed that women who restricted their milk and Vitamin D intake had lower birth weight babies.

Although low carbohydrate diets are the latest fad this is not the time for you to restrict carbohydrates. The recommended dietary allowance (RDA) for carbohydrates during pregnancy is 65% of total calories. This will help prevent you and your baby from suffering from low blood sugar. Low carbohydrate diets also can make it difficult for you to obtain certain necessary vitamins and minerals.

The March of Dimes, in an attempt to prevent spinal cord defects in unborn children, recommends that women who are trying to get pregnant should get *400 micrograms (mcg)* of folic acid, (a B vitamin), by eating fortified breakfast cereals, orange juice, beans, leafy green vegetables and a daily vitamin. Once you are pregnant they recommend 600 mcg and even more than this if there is a history of a prior neural tube defect (spina bifida).

Around the seventh or eight week of conception
your baby's heartbeat can be detected by ultrasound.
The heart beats between 40 – 80 times per minute
and it will double in size this week.
It is so large that it actually
"bulges" forward – not unlike a pregnant tummy.

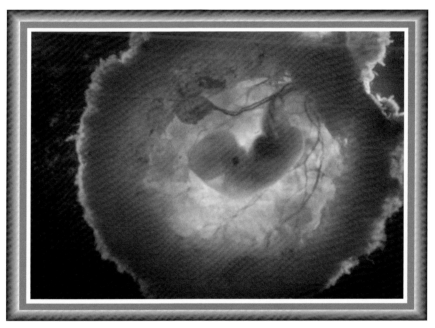

Photo: ©Claude Edelmann / Photo Researchers, Inc. 2006

Your healthcare provider will place you on prenatal vitamins to ensure that you receive the recommended vitamins and minerals that are necessary during your pregnancy. You should take them daily. However, they are not a replacement for a healthy diet.

TELLING THE BOSS

Although you may have told family and friends about your pregnancy, telling your boss is a different matter. Many women wait until the first trimester passes, knowing that the chance of miscarriage is higher during this period. Some women just tell their employers right away. When you decide to tell your employer is up to you.

There is no hard-and-fast rule. It depends a lot on what your position is within the organization, how long you have been with the company and how difficult it will be to replace you during your maternity leave. It's okay to wait but don't wait until you start showing. Also, your boss shouldn't hear this via the water-cooler grapevine. When you tell your boss be sure to have a plan of action ready for him with regards to how long you plan to work, how much family leave you will need and your suggestions for your replacement.

"Furnish an example, stop preaching, stop shielding, don't prevent self-reliance and initiative, allow your children to develop along their own lines."

– Eleanor Roosevelt

AT 10 WEEKS

By the end of the 10th week of your pregnancy all organs are represented and nearly all major structures are now formed. For the rest of your pregnancy your baby's development will consist of growing in size.

The sitting height of your unborn child is now about one inch, and its weight is about 0.1 ounce. The foot is 0.11 inch in length. Ultrasound measurement of sitting height (crown-rump length) can predict your due date within two days!

At this time, the fetal tail disappears. Its head continues to dominate its size. The fingers and toes become completely separated. The eyes are still far apart at this point, but the fetus is able to squint them. The eyelids and external ear are more completely developed. Taste buds begin and the nose remains plugged. By the end of the week, tooth buds of all twenty nonpermanent teeth will be present. If your fetus is a boy, its testes are already producing the male hormone, testosterone.

"All that I am my mother made me."

– John Quincy Adams

This is a side view of an embryo reconstructed graphically from a micro-MRI
at the end of the eighth week of development.
The lungs are the central structures of the respiratory system
and begin to form in the middle of the fourth week of development.
By the fifty-sixth day of development,
the right and left lobes of the lungs of the embryo have formed,
as well as branches of the bronchi.

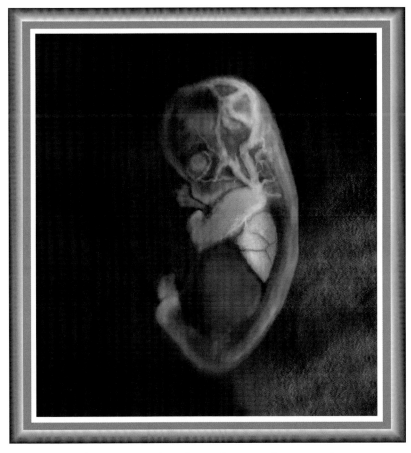

Photo: ©Anatomical Travelogue / Photo Researchers, Inc. 2006

Around the seventh or eighth week your unborn baby measures about
0.3 of an inch. The embryo's head, which is still bent onto the chest, is much
larger now and will grow even more to accommodate its rapidly enlarging brain.
Arm buds are now larger than leg buds and there is an obvious tail.
The backbone is now formed and the embryo's skin is so thin
that it is actually transparent. *A face is beginning to appear.*

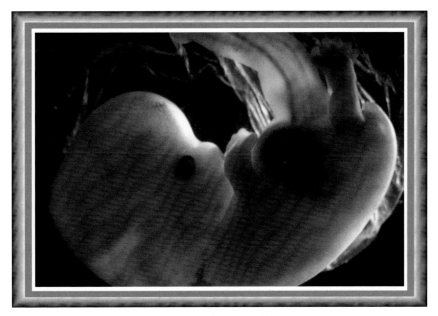

Photo: ©Petit Format / Photo Researchers, Inc. 2006

THE INEVITABLE WEIGHT GAIN

When women discover they are pregnant they become concerned with the inevitable body image changes that will occur. Many feel that all the hard work they have done to maintain a healthy weight and figure is going to go down the drain because of the pregnancy. Well if you are in good physical condition, congratulate yourself. This will make your pregnancy and delivery easier and you can continue with most exercise programs that you routinely do. For those of you who don't have a regular physical activity routine this would be a great time to start a walking program. It will help maintain energy levels, relieve indigestion and constipation, maintain a healthy weight gain and at the end of nine months help ease your delivery.

Eating well during pregnancy is vital but it does not give you permission to have a free for all. A balanced diet and monitoring your calorie intake is vital to your health and your baby's. During your first trimester you may experience nausea and vomiting. Constipation can cause you to feel bloated and full. This can make you feel like not eating and you might actually lose a couple of pounds at this time. During this trimester it is important to drink lots of water, eat a high-fiber diet and keep up your nutrition as best you can.

During the second trimester and third trimester you can expect to see a one pound weekly weight gain. Women who were underweight at the beginning of their pregnancy should see more and overweight women should see

"It is not a bad thing that children should occasionally and politely, put parents in their place."

– Colette

slightly less. The second trimester will bring relief from the chronic nausea and constipation. During your third trimester you may find yourself feeling full quickly and constipated again as your enlarging baby presses up on your stomach and intestines.

If the baby only weighs about 7.5 pounds where does all that weight go? According to the American College of Obstetricians and Gynecologists the rest of that weight is found in the amniotic fluid, placenta, uterus, breasts, body fluids, blood and maternal stores of fat, protein, and other nutrients.

This is not the time to try to lose or maintain your weight. You are expected to gain weight during pregnancy. It is part of what adds to the wonderful glow of pregnancy.

> "Thou art thy mother's glass, and she in thee Calls back the lovely April of her prime."
>
> – William Shakespeare

FETAL MAINTENANCE

It is grossly unfair to call the *placenta* merely "afterbirth," because it is one of the most remarkable organs in nature. During intrauterine life, it functions for the fetus as lung, liver, digestive tract, kidney and endocrine organ. And like the fetus, the placenta grows during pregnancy.

The placenta's physical structure is like a "blood filled sandwich." There is a mother's side and a baby's side to it with 12 to 20 blood-filled compartments in between, called "cotyledons." Along the floor of the mother's side, there are numerous holes and each one represents the opening of a small artery which squirts blood in a nozzle-like fashion. From the baby's side, hundreds of tree-like villi are suspended. Within these villi are the baby's capillaries across which the exchange of nutrients, wastes and oxygen takes place, but the mother's and fetus's blood do not mix. Placental development is necessary for the growth and well-being of the fetus.

THE UPS AND DOWNS

Have you noticed that your emotions seem to go from one extreme to the other? It's a beautiful weekend and you are resting in a chaise lounge on the porch watching a robin look for worms. You feel the warmth of the sun on your face, flowers are blooming and it's a great day. Unfortunately, thinking about how hard that poor robin has to work to find food has brought on a sudden outburst of tears and you find yourself crying uncontrollably. You feel like your heart is just breaking in two. But wait five minutes and you'll find the whole situation enormously funny and won't be able to stop the giggles. What is going on!? You're pregnant.

Hormonal changes, physical changes and psychological changes are intense right now, particularly during the first trimester. You are producing large amounts of hormones which can cause nausea and vomiting, breast tenderness and fatigue. Your sleep may be more restless and your dreams more intense. In fact you might even be having nightmares. Don't

"The hand that rocks the cradle Is the hand that rules the world."

– William Ross Wallace

worry, dreams are typically just a way for our brains to express anxiety that we feel over our changing bodies and developing pregnancy. They are probably intensified by the increased hormones.

You might be craving more physical affection from your mate. This is natural and a great opportunity to explore your physical relationship. Sex during pregnancy is safe and women often find their orgasms are more intense. If you both don't take yourselves too seriously it can be fun to explore different positions as your body grows.

The up and down feelings that you are experiencing are normal. If you find yourself feeling depressed for extended periods (greater than 2 weeks) talk to your physician. You may be clinically depressed and this is a treatable condition. Otherwise know that very soon, things will settle down. Try to enjoy that robin as often as you can.

Between seven and eight weeks the cells that will become sperm or eggs
now reach the ridge that represents the developing ovary or testes.
The long migration of these cells from yolk sac is complete.
The yolk sac (brown ball in upper right corner)
will now begin to break away and eventually disappear.

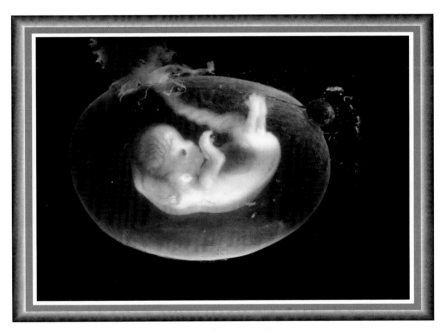

Photo: ©G. Moscoso / Photo Researchers, Inc. 2006

Between 8-10 weeks the genitalia will develop.

This is the beginning of the male genitalia.

The main swelling will develop into a penis over the coming weeks

and a scrotal sac will emerge.

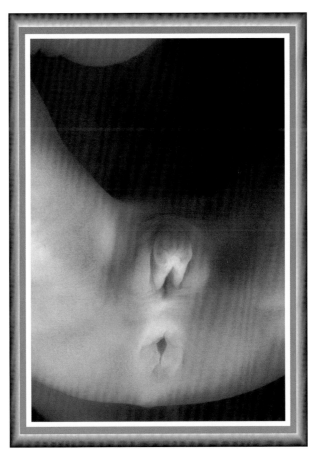

Photo: ©Neil Bromhall / Photo Researchers, Inc. 2006

This illustration of blood flow through a human placenta
shows the fetus next to a diagram of red blood cells
flowing through part of the placenta.
The irregular structure at the center is a chorionic villus
— a projection of fetal tissue into the maternal part of the placenta.
Deoxygenated blood (purple cells) from the fetus flows through this,
and picks up oxygenated blood cells (red) from the nearby maternal blood.
Arrows show direction of flow.
If some of the fetal blood cells (blue outline)
were to pass through the membrane into the maternal bloodstream,
they could cause hemolytic disease in the infant
if the mother is Rh negative and the baby is Rh positive.

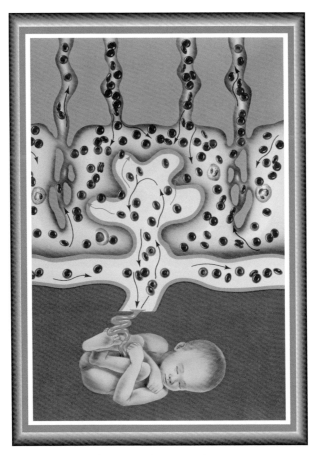

Photo: ©John Bavosi / Photo Researchers, Inc. 2006

This shows the lifeline (the umbilical cord),
connecting your baby (at the abdomen) with the placenta,
whose blood vessels are seen in the background.
The role of the placenta is complex:
apart from acting as an interface between the fetal & maternal circulations
(filtering & exchanging nourishment & waste products),
the placenta may be considered as a
multiple organ system for the developing fetus.

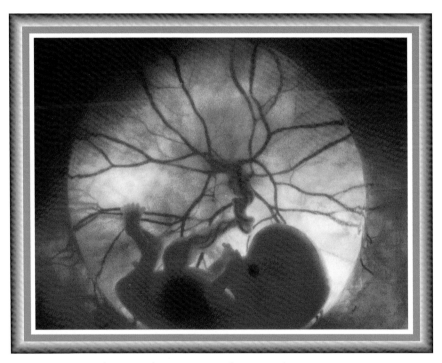

Photo: ©Nestle / Petit Format / Photo Researchers, Inc. 2006

The head is still relatively larger than the remainder of the body. Eyelids almost cover the eyes and the jaws are completely formed. External ears and a nose tip are now distinguishable.

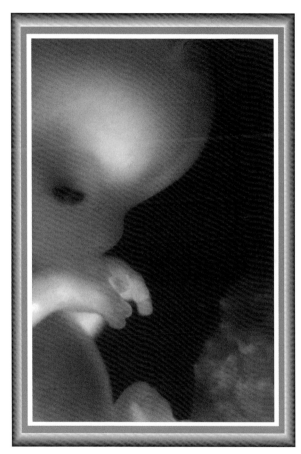

Photo: ©Petit Format / Photo Researchers, Inc. 2006

11 TO 12 WEEKS

The fetal head is more rounded now, but still so large that it represents almost one-half of its entire being. The eyelids are closing and will not reopen until the seventh to eighth month of pregnancy. The heart is now beating between 110 and 160 beats per minute. The intestines are still in the umbilical cord.

Growth remains rapid and for the first time the tiny fetal head is erect. Your fetus is now capable of spontaneous whole body movements. But these movements are only primitive reflexes; the brain is not yet developed enough to regulate them and won't be until after birth. Fingers and toes now have nails and even some hair is present. The profile of the face is now distinctly human.

> "Life began with waking up and loving my mother's face. . . ."
>
> – George Eliot

The big hernia opening into the umbilical cord will correct itself during this week, so that the intestines return into the baby's abdominal cavity. The pancreas can now manufacture insulin.

For the first time, it is possible to distinguish by external appearance whether your fetus is a boy or girl. If the fetus is a boy, the female system (which would have developed into a uterus, tubes and vagina) has disappeared.

The amount of amniotic fluid now present in the "bag of waters" is between 3 and 4 tablespoons. The uterus, now about 3 to 4 inches in diameter, is too big to stay in the pelvis and rises into your abdominal cavity. It can usually be felt by your healthcare provider just above the pubic hairline.

WHEW! FIRST TRIMESTER IS DONE

You have just completed your first trimester. One-third of your pregnancy is over! Your embryo became a fetus and your child has completely developed all of the necessary organs, limbs and features that make him/her distinct. The first bone tissue has appeared and ribs are distinguishable. His/Her nose and chin are now quite distinct. Movement becomes more pronounce and your baby can even suck his/her thumb!

Ultrasounds have been able to detect breathing-like movements at this early stage, although actual breathing does not start until after birth. The lips are able to open and close and a primitive circulation takes place. The fetus swallows amniotic fluid and excretes it back as urine.

By now you have probably gained about two pounds. Your heart beat has increased slightly (about 4 to 8 beats per minute faster than usual) to accommodate the increase in blood volume. Your body has gone through some of the most remarkable changes it will ever experience in these last three months. You are truly the caretaker of the generations.

"The most important thing a father can do for his children is to love their mother."

– Author Unknown

Congratulations!

You have just finished your first trimester of pregnancy.

Keep reading! There is a lot more excitement ahead.

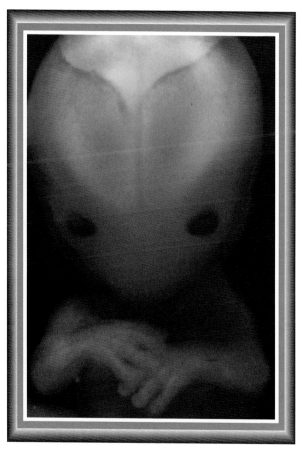

Photo: ©Petit Format / Photo Researchers, Inc. 2006

THE SECOND TRIMESTER

"Before you were conceived I wanted you

Before you were born I loved you

Before you were here an hour I would die for you

This is the miracle of life."

—Maureen Hawkins

This is your baby around week 14. Cheeks are developing and movement becomes regular. In a couple of more weeks you will most likely experience those movements as butterflies in your tummy At fourteen weeks your baby's arms and legs are well differentiated. The skin is very thin and transparent.

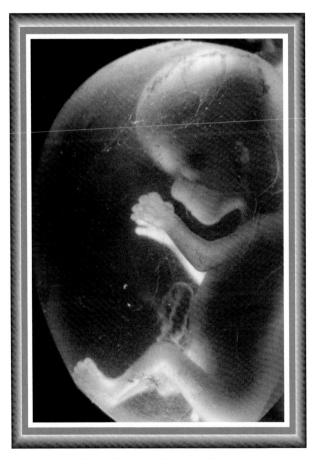

Photo: ©Claude Edelmann / Photo Researchers, Inc. 2006

*Y*our second trimester has begun. Your unborn baby is experiencing continued growth of its organ systems and body. You are finally starting to feel better and the nausea, vomiting, breast tenderness and fatigue of the last trimester are beginning to fade. This is when people start to notice the "glow" of your pregnancy. You feel good, you will begin to "show" as your baby grows and your emotions become your own again. This is the trimester when any moving, traveling or even surgery should be done.

> "We worry about what a child will become tomorrow, yet we forget that he is someone today."
>
> – Stacia Tauscher

THE MYSTERY OF GENETICS

This is the time when your healthcare provider will determine whether you need an *amniocentesis* by reviewing your risk factors. Things like your family history (any congenital defects or Down's syndrome), your age and your exposure to potential toxins will influence the decision. Sometimes your healthcare provider may have you seek genetic counseling. Genetic counseling can determine your potential risk, outline possible plans of action and communicate with your obstetrician the need for amniocentesis or other testing.

In most instances your amniocentesis will be normal and offer you a great deal of reassurance. If defects are discovered, you will be armed with information and can begin to make preparations at home and within the family for the event of this birth. This information also allows physicians to prepare and plan what will be needed for pregnancy, labor, delivery and postpartum care.

The most common test, amniocentesis, is a test of the amniotic fluid. It detects chromosomal abnormalities such as Down's syndrome, spinal cord defects, and several *X-linked disorders* (which means they are handed down from the female side of either parent) such as *hemophilia*. Amniocentesis can also detect the sex of the fetus, but physicians will rarely perform the procedure for that reason alone.

There is another test that can be done, usually towards the end of the first trimester called *chorionic villous* sampling. This test takes a small biopsy of the placenta, usually by going through the cervix. It is able to detect genetic abnormalities but it does not pick up on *neural tube defects* (spinal cord defects). There are also blood and cell tests that can detect about sixty or so chromosomal and other disorders.

Obviously, these tests are looking for genetic disorders, problems that you don't have any control over. But there are things that you can do to protect your unborn child from birth defects. You will want to get enough sleep and eat right. As soon as you announce your pregnancy, friends and family will have their own recommendations as to how to do the best by your unborn child. Endure this with a smile (they have the best of intentions), but there are some specific danger zones that you should be aware of.

"It will be gone before you know it. The fingerprints on the wall appear higher and higher. Then suddenly they disappear."

– Dorothy Evslin

DANGER ZONES

First and foremost, if you are smoking, QUIT! You are literally suffocating your child. Smoking during pregnancy has been linked to premature births, uterine growth restriction, attention deficit disorder, math and language problems and auditory processing difficulties. Worse yet it has been linked to sudden infant death. This applies to exposure to second hand smoke as well. Stay away from smokers.

Alcohol abuse is a well studied addiction that can lead to fetal alcohol syndrome. You might say "I'm not addicted or abusing alcohol" but the problem with this reasoning is we don't know how much alcohol it takes to harm an unborn child. Fetal Alcohol Syndrome can produce babies who are born early and are very underweight, have difficulty eating or sleeping, have problems learning or paying attention, or have heart defects and may need medical care all of their lives. Some may die before they are born. The American College of Obstetricians and Gynecologists recommends that if you drink, stop! If you have an addiction, seek help from your physician.

So called recreational drugs are another problem for your fetus. Do you really want your baby smoking pot? If you are smoking, your baby is smoking.

One of the most disturbing sounds heard in a neonatal nursery is the scream of a newborn that has been exposed to cocaine use during its mother's pregnancy. These babies are addicted, underweight, have severe

"Children are the living messages we send to a time we will not see."

– John W. Whitehead, *The Stealing of America,* 1983

developmental disorders and do not sleep or eat well. Crystal meth can also cause enduring cognitive deficits that can never be reversed. If you are using, stop immediately! Your baby's life depends on it.

These are specific danger zones that women in their reproductive years can be exposed to. Protect your unborn baby by eating right, sleeping well and stay away from substances that could potentially ruin your baby's life forever.

WHEN YOU KNOW IT ISN'T GAS!

By now, you have probably felt the first signs of "quickening," the first sensation of your unborn baby's movements. This usually occurs sometime between 16 and 20 weeks because the amniotic fluid has significantly increased and your baby's size has enlarged. Movement within the fluid feels a little like butterflies in the belly. It is so exciting the first time you notice quickening. It might be just a brief sensation and you don't pay much attention the first time, but then it happens again. You *know* that's your baby! For many women, quickening is a time when significant bonding begins with the baby. This is when you begin to comprehend daily, that there is a life within you. Now, when you go to work, watch TV, or go about other daily routines, you understand that you have along a tiny partner that is growing and changing every day.

"A woman with a child rediscovers the world. All is changed — politics, loyalties, needs. For now all is judged by the life of the child . . . and of all children."

– Pam Brown

Your baby's face now *has cheeks* at 16 weeks. Its eyes are beginning to appear more forward in the head, rather than on the side, and the eyelids remain closed. The bridge of its nose is now seen, and a downy type of hair called *lanugo* is present. The fetus's head becomes erect and its legs become longer than its arms during this trimester. Fingernails become well developed, too. The ears stand out from the head, and the fetus now has the same number of nerve cells as an adult.

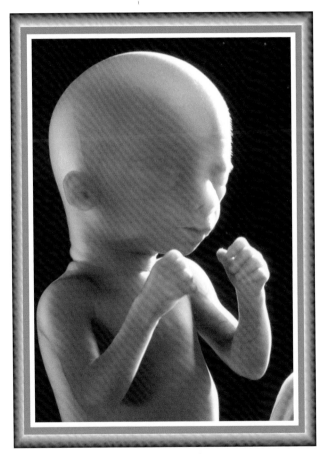

Photo: ©Tissuepix / Photo Researchers, Inc. 2006

YOUR BABY IS GROWING RAPIDLY

Your little partner is developing quickly. Since your unborn baby's physical structure was developed and put into place during the first trimester, now, and in the weeks to come, this structure increases in both length, weight, and density. In this trimester, the diameter of the fetal head can be measured by ultrasound and an estimate of the duration of pregnancy can be calculated from this measurement. At this stage of pregnancy, breathing, sucking and swallowing are all possible. The fetus is also capable of frowning and opening its mouth.

Your baby's face now has cheeks. Its eyes are beginning to appear more forward in the head, rather than on the side, and the eyelids remain closed. The eyes will move forward even more this trimester, but there is still a wide space between them. The bridge of its nose is now seen, and a downy type of hair called *lanugo* is present. The fetus's head becomes erect and its legs become longer than its arms during this trimester. Fingernails become well developed, too. The ears stand out from the head, and the fetus now has the same number of nerve cells as an adult. The retinas of the eyes become sensitive to light. By week 23 your unborn child will be sufficiently developed so that he/she is able to suck, and eyebrows will be well developed.

"In the sheltered simplicity of the first days after a baby is born, one sees again the magical closed circle, the miraculous sense of two people existing only for each other."

– Anne Morrow Lindbergh

TINY BEATS

The fetal heart now pumps at 117 to 157 beats per minute. Research has shown that a fetus born at this age has a pattern of waves on an electrocardiogram (EKG) that is similar to an adult's. The fetal heart is now large enough that it can be heard with the aid of a Doppler probe. A Doppler is a small device that amplifies the sound of blood flow within the vessels. It can detect your baby's heartbeat, amplify it and then transmit it through a speaker so that you and your healthcare provider can hear it.

"You can fool all of the people some of the time, and some of the people all of the time, but you can't fool Mom."

– Unknown

GENITALS

If female, the fetus's ovaries descend from the abdomen into the fetal pelvis. If male, the prostate gland is now first seen. If your fetus is male, his scrotum will still be solid at this stage, but if female, the fetus's vagina begins to hollow out. The female fetus has approximately six million eggs by now, but even this early in its development, the fetus's eggs start to disappear by some still mysterious process of degeneration. By the time of birth, the number of eggs will be reduced to about one million. During a woman's reproductive life, only 300 to 400 will mature and be released (one each month) as potential candidates for fertilization by sperm. At the end of this trimester, sexual organ differentiation will be complete.

Your baby at about the 4th month of development, showing the head & upper limbs & the umbilical cord which connects the fetus (at the navel) to the placenta. There is a lot of room within the uterus and amniotic fluid right now, so the baby just floats freely. Growth at this time is rapid: the head is still relatively large with a bulging forehead, the outer ear is formed, as are the nose & mouth, and the eyes have migrated from the sides of the head. Forearms, wrists, hands & fingers are well differentiated, developing at a faster rate than the lower limbs.

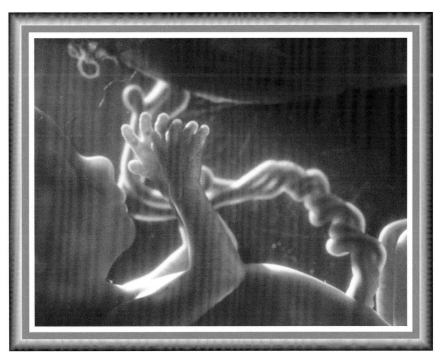

Photo: ©Nestle / Petit Format / Photo Researchers, Inc. 2006

During this trimester your baby will be growing in size,
adding fat and developing skills, such as learning how to suck his/her thumb!

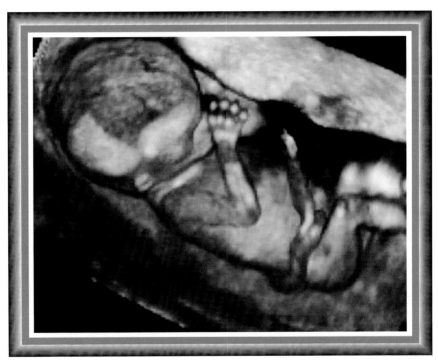

Photo: ©GE Medical Systems / Photo Researchers, Inc. 2006

The fetal skeleton continues to produce more bone.

Enough now that it can be seen by x-ray.

Previously they contained too little calcium to be seen.

The arms can bend at the elbows and wrists.

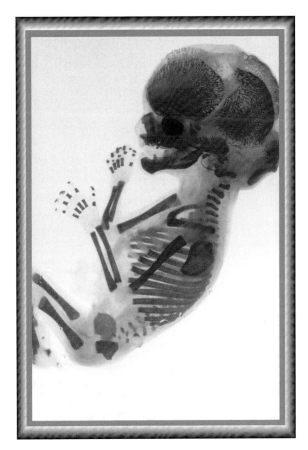

Photo: ©Biophoto Associates / Photo Researchers, Inc. 2006

BABY GYM

The fetal skeleton continues to produce more bone. The arms can bend at the elbows and wrists. Fetal fingers can close tightly to form fists but none of these movements are as yet controlled by the brain; they are reflexive only. Parts of the fetal skeleton can now be seen by x-ray. Previously they contained too little calcium to be visible by that means. Stretching movements of the arms and legs can be seen by ultrasound! By week 22 your unborn child will be able to react to loud noises or to music! Does this represent exercise? We don't really know. But it's fun to think about our little fetus doing aerobics inside the uterus. He or she begins to have alternating periods of sleep and wakefulness, and a tap on mother's abdomen can awaken a sleeping fetus.

> "Anyone who thinks the art of conversation is dead ought to tell a child to go to bed."
>
> – Robert Gallagher

BREATHING PRACTICE

Respiratory-type movements of the fetus's chest can be detected. The fetus can move amniotic fluid into and out of the lungs, about a pint a day it is thought, and excretes a similar amount through fetal urine. Although the fetus both swallows and breathes amniotic fluid, true gas exchange – the essence of respiration – does not occur until the air sacs of the lungs expand. This expansion cannot take place until a baby takes its first breath. Since the lungs do not function as an organ of respiration until delivery, the fetus can "breathe" fluid without drowning. The small amount of fluid present in the lungs at the time of delivery is simply absorbed. Swallowing and breathing require complex coordination between nerves and muscles. Amniotic fluid provides a good "practice" medium for this activity before birth.

WAXING UP

Special glands in the fetus's skin are actively making a waxy coating, called *vernix*. This skin coating allows unborn babies to float in the amniotic fluid for several months without skin damage. The fetus's skin is getting thicker and is no longer transparent. At this time, too, a special kind of heat-regulating fat, called *brown fat* is first seen. *Lanugo* now covers its entire body, and some scalp hair is present as well. Toenails begin to form. By week 24, fat begins to build up under the skin but the fetus as a whole is still quite lean.

YOUR BABY HAS GROWN

At the end of this trimester your unborn baby will be about 9.2 inches (sitting height) in length and weigh about 2 pounds, 3 ounces. If measured by ultrasound, the diameter of its head will be 6.7 centimeters. For the remainder of the pregnancy, this measurement becomes a less accurate predictor of due date; it can only predict it within a two week time span.

"Making the decision to have a child – it's momentous. It is to decide forever to have your heart go walking around outside your body."

– Elizabeth Stone

WALK, TWO, THREE, FOUR!

You are going to experience significant changes during this trimester too. The greatest weight gain for most women takes place now in the second trimester as fat storage begins. Most women are now gaining approximately one pound per week. The nausea of the first trimester has usually subsided and your appetite is increased. This increase is a natural response to the changes in your metabolism and allows you to consume the 300 to 600 extra calories daily that your body needs.

As an active woman who exercises regularly you may have some concerns about continuing your exercise program during your pregnancy. The American College of Obstetricians and Gynecologists (ACOG) have studied this issue and have several recommendations. First they acknowledge that 30 minutes or more of moderate exercise a day should occur on most if not all days of the week in the absence of either medical or obstetrical complications for optimum health maintenance. Data has been published that suggests exercise is also beneficial in preventing gestational diabetes. Women who exercise regularly during their pregnancies usually have an easier time during labor and delivery, less indigestion and heartburn, and more energy.

In general, ACOG feels that participation in most recreational activities is safe. They do advise avoiding activities such as hockey, soccer, basketball, downhill skiing, racquet sports,

> "You may have tangible wealth untold;
> Caskets of jewels and coffers of gold.
> Richer than I you can never be –
> I had a mother who read to me."
>
> – Strickland Gillian

horseback riding, and waterskiing due to potential high impact around the abdominal area. Most women who are pregnant can continue to jog (if they were jogging prior to pregnancy), bicycle, walk, yoga, Pilates and any other moderate intensity activity that does not involve high impact contact.

"Becoming a mother makes you the mother of all children. From now on each wounded, abandoned, frightened child is yours. You live in the suffering mothers of every race and creed and weep with them. You long to comfort all who are desolate."

– Charlotte Gray

You may experience some shortness of breath or even lightheadedness when you exert yourself or exercise. Generally this is caused by a decrease in your blood pressure which results from the enlarged uterus pressing on, and therefore constricting, major blood vessels. Therefore it is important to avoid doing exercises that call for prolonged periods of lying on your back.

ACOG recommends immediate cessation of any exercise if any one of these warning signs are present: vaginal bleeding, dizziness, headache, chest pain, muscle weakness, calf pain or swelling, contractions, decreased fetal movement or amniotic fluid leakage. You should immediately report any of the above to your healthcare provider.

The slowing down of maternal blood circulation often causes muscle cramps, especially in the legs. For women susceptible to them, such cramps seem to be worse at night or in cold weather. Some women find that an increase in their daily intake of calcium helps to alleviate these cramps. Elevating the legs and use of a heating pad also aid in lessening such discomfort.

This colored ultrasound photograph captured this baby blowing bubbles.
He/She can move amniotic fluid into and out of the lungs, about a pint a day,
and excretes a similar amount through fetal urine.
Although the fetus both swallows and breathes amniotic fluid,
true gas exchange – the essence of respiration – does not occur until
the air sacs of the lungs expand at birth.

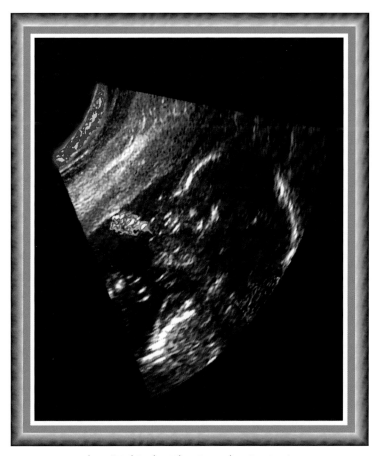

Photo: ©Neil Borden / Photo Researchers, Inc. 2006

HEARTBURN, INDIGESTION, CONSTIPATION; OH MY!

Indigestion and heartburn are frequent occurrences now and through the duration of pregnancy. These discomforts have several causes. First, there has been an increase in the production of the progesterone hormone in the mother's system. This hormone delays the emptying of the stomach and retards the closing activity between the stomach and the esophagus. The delay results in a backup of acids and digestive juices from the stomach into the esophagus, causing heartburn.

Also, the growth of the fetus and uterus push upward and displace the stomach. The mother's diaphragm rises almost two inches and her lower ribs spread outward. This upward movement adds to the feelings of indigestion and heartburn as well.

A simple technique to help avoid the heartburn and indigestion is to eat smaller meals more frequently throughout the day. Your stomach won't be as full and there will be less to digest.

The increased amount of progesterone that the mother's body produces serves to relax all smooth muscles, but this can make her bowels (which are also smooth muscles), less efficient and constipation can result. This is why it is important to get regular exercise and eat a diet high in fiber.

"The mother love is like God's love; He loves us not because we are lovable, but because it is His nature to love, and because we are His children."

– Earl Riney

YOU MAY NOT NEED *VICTORIA'S SECRET*

Significant swelling and enlargement of the breasts can begin from the outset of pregnancy. For some women this is an opportunity to enjoy an increased sense of ampleness and sexuality. The enlargement is caused by the development of milk glands and hormone stimulation. The average increase in breast size is about 200 millimeters (one cup size) for each breast. The nipple also increases in size as well. Soreness and tenderness often accompany this enlargement as well as a darkening in the area around the nipples.

Sometimes a watery, sticky fluid will be secreted from the nipples, although this usually happens later in pregnancy for most women. Using some type of emollient cream will help keep the tenderness to a minimum.

"Before becoming a mother I had a hundred theories on how to bring up children. Now I have seven children and only one theory: love them, especially when they least deserve to be loved."

- Kate Samperi

FOREIGN AFFAIRS

By week 20, your uterus will have grown large enough to reach your navel because of the baby's growth and placental growth. The placenta now weighs 8 to 9 ounces. The placenta — and, for that matter, the baby itself — is really "foreign" tissue to the mother's body. The baby and the placenta arise from genes of both its mother and father. Because the father's tissue is now growing within the mother's uterus, this new tissue (baby, placenta and membranes) is really a transplant. If so, why doesn't rejection take place? Or is labor itself the end-product of a slow, on-going "rejection" process? The answer to this riddle may well solve current questions about the rejection problems involved with organ transplants; and there is current, active research in this area.

This beautiful photo of a fetus at 19 weeks shows this baby sucking the thumb surrounded by the transparent membranes of the amniotic sac.

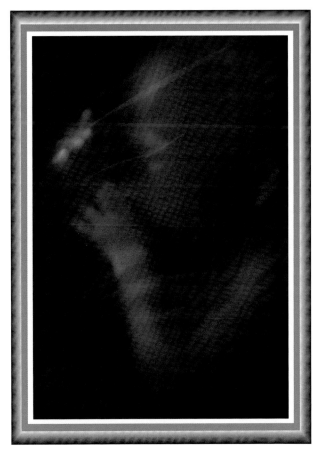

Photo: ©Bromhall / Photo Researchers, Inc. 2006

At 20 weeks the eyelids are well formed and will stay closed until around the third trimester. The eyes will move forward even more, for there is still a wide space between them. The retinas of the eyes become sensitive to light.

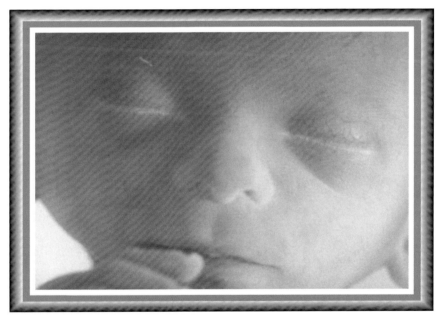

Photo: ©Petit Format / Photo Researchers, Inc. 2006

OTHER CHANGES

A mother's skin, too, may undergo changes during pregnancy. In two out of three Caucasian women and about 10 percent of African-American women, so-called "spiders" – tiny red marks on the face, shoulders and arms – develop. These are caused by local dilation of blood vessels and usually disappear after delivery.

About two-thirds of Caucasian women and one out of three African-American women develop a reddening of their palms. The appearance of brown spots on the face neck and abdomen, showing as white spots on women of color, are known as the "mask of pregnancy." These, too, usually disappear in the month after delivery.

There is a marked increase in your blood volume and increased output of blood from your heart by this stage of pregnancy. This increased blood volume exerts pressure on the small capillaries found in the lining of the nose and the gums. This pressure is enough to produce spontaneous nosebleeds or bleeding gums. Lubricating the nostrils with petroleum jelly can alleviate the nosebleeds; while a diet rich in protein, calcium and vitamins C, B, and D can prevent teeth and gum problems. Be sure to see your dentist regularly throughout your pregnancy.

Like so many other organs in her body, a mother's thyroid gland is more active during pregnancy. One result of this increased activity can be a tendency to perspire more heavily than usual. A mother's body also generates more heat during pregnancy. In order to maintain a normal temperature, perspiration or sweating

"The strength of motherhood is greater than natural laws."

– Barbara Kingsolver

increases. This mechanism also allows the body to rid itself, through perspiration, of excessive waste products that build up during pregnancy.

The increase in body temperature that most women experience can make the expectant mother uncomfortable, especially during summer months, but even in winter, it's advisable to avoid excess clothing and to use body powder or cornstarch to absorb perspiration and thereby avoid chafing and skin irritations.

Again, due to the increased production of progesterone during pregnancy, a woman's gallbladder does not empty well so there is an increased chance of gallstones. Although it is unusual for the condition to become severe enough to warrant surgery, (should it be necessary), the second trimester is considered safe for surgery for both mother and baby.

DONE WITH ANOTHER TRIMESTER!

Congratulations — another trimester is complete. You are now two-thirds through your pregnancy. Your baby has developed all his organs and body structures, he/she has put on weight and size and you have been getting compliments about how beautiful you look because you are taking good care of yourself. It's time for the final three.

During this trimester your baby's fingernails become well developed, too. The ears
stand out from the head,
and your little partner becomes very distinctly human.

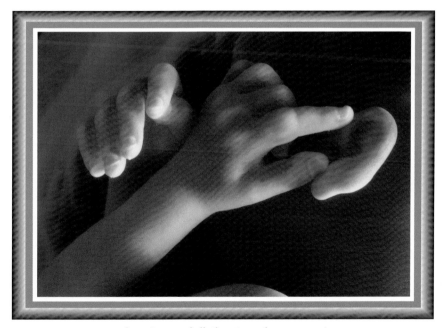

Photo: ©N. Bromhall/PhotoResearchers, Inc. 2006

At 20 weeks your baby is very thin, has very little fat underneath the skin,
and is covered by lanugo (downy hair).
Until he gets more time in the womb he will remain red and wrinkled.

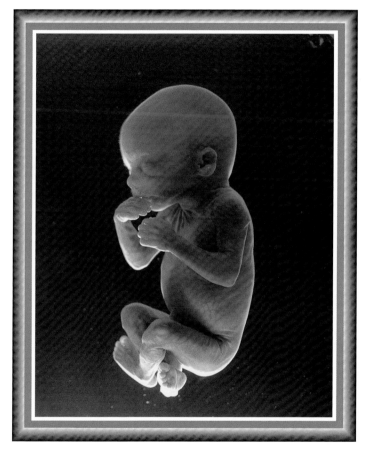

Photo: ©James Stevenson /Photo Researchers, Inc. 2006

This fetus is about 24 weeks young.
You can see how transparent and thin the baby's skin remains
at this point in its development.

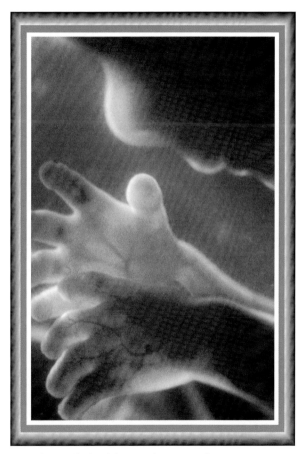

Photo: ©Claude Edelmann / Photo Researchers, Inc. 2006

THE THIRD TRIMESTER

"God could not be everywhere,
and therefore He created mothers."
—Jewish Proverb

Things are starting to get a little cramped inside the womb.
This sleeping baby seems so content in his limited space.
Perhaps that's why babies find such security in being "wrapped"
in their blankets when they are born.

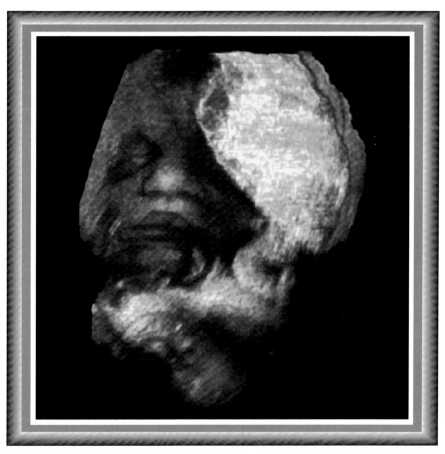

Photo: ©Siemens Ultrasound 2006

*N*ow things are getting really exciting! You have just finished your second trimester and you are in the home stretch. This is when the real fun begins; designing the baby's room, buying baby clothes, going to baby showers, and Lamaze classes, choosing baby names and picking out birth announcements. Your prenatal care visits will become more frequent and your tummy is going to get more rounded as baby grows. You should be experiencing frequent fetal movement and, by the end of this trimester, may even be able to identify a foot or hand as your baby moves around inside you.

OLD WIVES' TALES

"My mother is my root, my foundation. She planted the seed that I base my life on, and that is the belief that the ability to achieve starts in your mind."

– Michael Jordan

You and your baby are continuing on the journey of growth and development and soon your child will become a viable infant. There is an old wives' tale which claims that a baby born prematurely in the seventh calendar month has a better chance of survival than one born in the eighth calendar month. Nothing could be more erroneous. Everyday a fetus gets closer to forty weeks, the greater its chances for survival. An infant that weighs less than five pounds (2500 grams) is considered premature. Such infants often have lungs that are too immature to perform the complexities of respiration. Fortunately, we have come a long way in caring for these very fragile preemies. Hospitals throughout the nation have special units designed just for these babies and there are doctors who specialize in the care of premature infants. Although by the time you reach your eighth month of pregnancy you may be wishing that labor would just start, remember that your child needs all that time in your body to develop strong lungs, musculature and bone mass.

REMEMBER, THERE ARE TWO OF YOU!

During this trimester, you will experience the greatest changes in your own body, both in size and mobility. The increased weight on the front of your body will throw off your normal balance and posture, requiring you to adopt a new stance. At this point your exercise routine may have to be adjusted. A regular 30-minute walk can continue to provide you with all the benefits of exercise; however, you might have to take it slower. Your increased weight will also make it difficult to find a comfortable sleeping position, to bend over, to fit behind a steering wheel and to find comfortable clothes. Backaches and swollen ankles are not uncommon. The good news is that these discomforts will soon be rewarded. In the meantime, you should remain focused on what the end results will be. Keep in mind what you are learning about your baby's development and growth inside you. Let that be where your thoughts are directed when you are feeling too bulky to carry on.

"Nothing else will ever make you a s happy or as sad, as proud or as tired, as motherhood."

— Elia Parsons

This artistic representation of your baby in the womb at the beginning of the last trimester shows you how far he/she has come since his/her conception. But your baby still needs to put on more weight and to mature its lungs prior to being born.

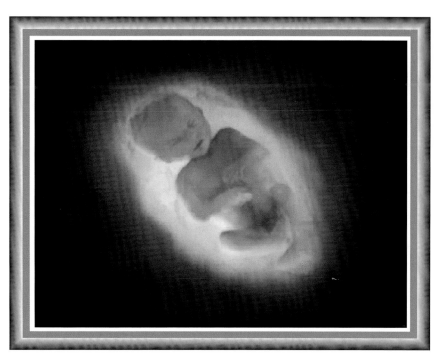

Photo: ©ICAM/Mona Lisa/Eurelios/Phototake 2006

SEAT BELTS

Speaking of fitting behind a steering wheel now is a good time to talk about seat belts. As a responsible person, you always use your seat belt. Now, however, you are worried about putting a seat belt across your expanding abdomen. In their September 1998 educational bulletin, the American College of Obstetricians and Gynecologists state that "there is substantial evidence that seat belt use during pregnancy protects both the mother and the fetus. Nonetheless, many pregnant women do not wear seat belts properly." Their recommendations are that both the lap belt and shoulder harness should be used. The lap belt is to be placed under the abdomen, over both hip bones and your pubic bone. The shoulder harness should be placed between the breasts. You do not need excessive slack in either belt; you should wear them as snugly as is comfortable. They also state that airbag deployment does not appear to be associated with increased risk for mother or baby. You do not have to disable your airbags while you are pregnant. So please, wear your seat belt properly each and every time you are in the car.

"The formative period for building character for eternity is in the nursery. The mother is queen of that realm and sways a scepter more potent than that of kings or priests."

– Author Unknown

TALK ABOUT BEING PUSHED AROUND . . .

If you think about it, the uterus is a remarkable organ. It increases at least tenfold in weight during pregnancy and increases at least 500 times in volume! By the end of pregnancy there has been a tremendous increase in weight of the mother's uterus. It will weigh about 2 pounds, 2 ounces. Prior to pregnancy it weighed about 2 ounces!

But, it is the expanding uterus that is pushing the intestines, stomach, and diaphragm higher. Your abdominal organs are being squeezed and pushed up against your diaphragm. Your stomach cannot expand after a meal like it use to. Such changes contribute to an increasing sense of fullness, bloating, indigestion and heartburn. Eating smaller more frequent meals throughout the day can help with these irritations.

> "Mother —
> that was the bank where we deposited all our hurts and worries."
>
> – T. DeWitt Talmage

BRAXTON HICKS

During this third trimester, many women experience periodic uterine contractions know as *Braxton Hicks* contractions. These are usually experienced as a tightening at the top of the uterus that spreads downward and then relaxes. Such contractions can sometimes be quite strong, but they are not frequent or at regular intervals, so they can be distinguished from the start of actual labor. During childbirth preparation classes, many women take advantage of such "trial" contractions to practice their breathing techniques. These contractions also serve to strengthen the uterus and often provide early dilation or effacement of your cervix before actual labor begins.

This is a colored 3-dimensional magnetic resonance imaging (MRI) scan
of a healthy fetus approaching full term.
The baby is facing towards the mother's back (left).
The umbilical cord is seen at center.
The baby's brain, spinal column, heart, liver and lungs are also visible.
Notice how close to the diaphragm the uterus is.

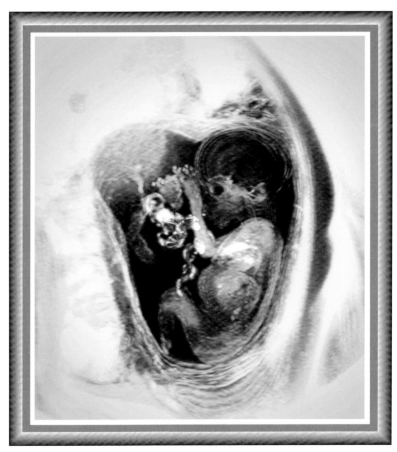

Photo: ©DuCane Medical Imaging Ltd. / Photo Researchers, Inc. 2006

As your baby continues to grow in this trimester both and you and he/she are going to start feeling like space is getting tight. Your baby will have less room to move around, although will probably be more active in this trimester and you will start to feel the effects of the baby's increasing size.

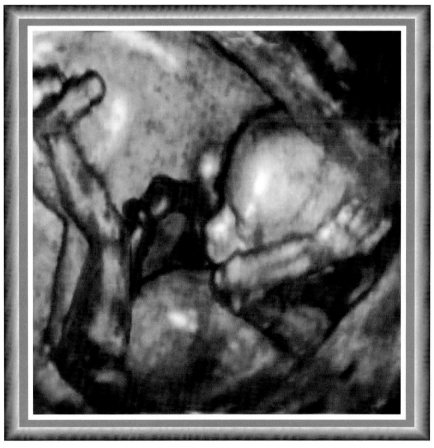

Photo: © GE Medical Systems / Photo Researchers, Inc. 2006

GETTING READY FOR BIRTH

As your due date gets closer, the fetus begins to "snuggle" into the pelvis in preparation for birth. The great majority of babies are born with a *cephalic* presentation, that is with the fetus's head leading and turned toward the mother's tailbone. However, in about 3 percent of deliveries, the baby is in a *breech* presentation with its legs in the bottom of the uterus in various positions. An even more rare presentation is *transverse,* where the baby is lying sideways in the uterus. Unless it can be moved into a cephalic position, a baby in such a position must be delivered by cesarean section.

WHERE DOES AMNIOTIC FLUID COME FROM?

The placenta now has a total surface area of 10 square meters! It weighs slightly more than one pound, measures about 8 inches in diameter, and is about 1 inch thick. This dramatic increase in size provides a large area for exchange of nutrients and waste products between you and your baby. He/She is surrounded by two sacs: the inner *amnion* and the outer *chorion.* The *chorion* is actually a sac around a sac, but the two sacs are so close that they appear as one "bag." The amniotic fluid is within these sacs, and together the sacs are referred to as "membranes." When the

"Bitter are the
tears of a child:
Sweeten them.
Deep are the thoughts of a child:
Quiet them.
Sharp is the grief of a child:
Take it from him.
Soft is the heart of a child:
Do not harden it."

– Pamela Glenconner

membranes are ruptured, usually during labor, the fused sacs are pierced and fluid is allowed to flow out the birth canal (vagina). Should these membranes rupture before labor, you should call your physician immediately.

The amniotic fluid the baby floats in comes from the prodigious exchange between mother and baby and fetal urine. By now there is about 2 pints of water in the amniotic sac. This entire amount is exchanged and replaced every two hours. As pregnancy progresses, the "placental barrier" between the mother's blood and the baby's blood vessels is very thin, only 0.002 millimeters (0.0008 inch) thick. An amazing amount of material is transferred in both directions. Water crosses the barrier in excess of 1 pint per second! Nature has built into it an incredible "margin of safety." It has been estimated that 99.9 percent of the water and salt that reaches the fetus is returned to the mother! Your baby also swallows slightly less than one pint of amniotic fluid each day. Then he/she produces between 25 and 30 milliliters (about 2 tablespoons) of urine per hour. This urine is passed into the amniotic fluid in which the fetus floats and, thus, accounts for about 650 milliliters (over 1 pint) of fluid per day.

The placenta receives a large amount of blood from both the fetus and its mother, but their blood never mixes. Fetal blood stays in vessels which are contained within structures called *villi* as mentioned earlier. The mother's blood

> "My mother's menu consisted of two choices: Take it or leave it."
>
> – Buddy Hackett

bathes a space called the *intervillous space*. The villi literally hang like branching tree limbs into this space and are bathed by mother's blood. Exchange of nutrients and waste products occur across the thin walls of the villi and the fetal blood vessels.

After delivery, you may want to see your placenta, or "afterbirth." It is truly a remarkable organ. The dull shaggy side is the surface that's attached to the uterus; while the shiny, gleaming side is the one from which the umbilical cord arises and represents the baby's side. The mother's side – the shaggy one – contains the compartments called *cotyledons*.

BANKING CORD BLOOD

The human species is the only one in which there is a large amount of blood – slightly more than one pint, lost at the time of delivery. Moments after birth, the newborn's circulation of blood is entirely different than that before birth. The reason is that before birth, the placenta did the work of the lungs, and a majority of fetal blood was able to bypass the lungs. After birth, these passages close and the entire infant's blood supply must then pass through its lungs for exchange of oxygen and carbon dioxide.

Cord blood also contains stem cells which research suggests will be the new wave of treatment for disease. Many women are now choosing to bank their baby's cord blood. A sterile sample of cord blood is obtained immediately after delivery, specially packaged and mailed to a company that will freeze and then store the sample. The sample is then kept until such time as it might be needed to treat you, your partner, your child or a sibling. The reason this works is because stem cells contain the building blocks necessary to become any cell within the body. When stimulated properly they have the potential to replace damaged heart cells, kidney cells and even liver cells. Stem cells may soon be used to treat Alzheimer's, Parkinson's, stroke, kidney failure, diabetes, heart attacks, immune deficiencies, Tay Sachs, testicular cancer, Hodgkin's, multiple myeloma, brain tumors and other devastating diseases.

"If you bungle raising your children, I don't think whatever else you do well matters very much."

– Jacqueline Kennedy Onassis

The reason to store your baby's cord blood is because the "match" rate will be closer to 100%. While there are compelling reasons to bank your baby's cord blood, it is expensive. The initial costs at one site were close to $2000 and, additionally, there is a yearly fee. Unfortunately, at the time of this writing, cord blood banking is not considered standard of care and, therefore, is not covered by insurance.

In this artistic rendition the baby is full-term. As your due date gets closer, the fetus begins to "snuggle" into the pelvis in preparation for birth. The great majority of babies are born with a *cephalic* presentation, that is with the fetus's head leading and turned toward the mother's tailbone.

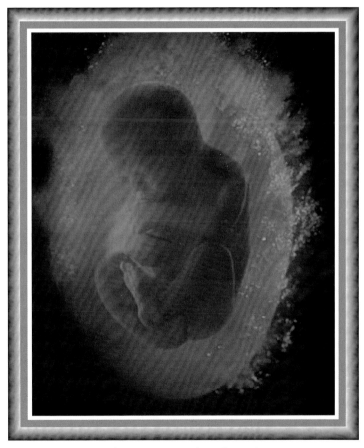

Photo: © Yoav Levy/Phototake 2006

After delivery, you may want to see your placenta, or "afterbirth."

It is truly a remarkable organ.

The dull shaggy side is the surface that's attached to the uterus;

while the shiny, gleaming side is the one from which

the umbilical cord arises and represents the baby's side.

The mother's side – the shaggy one –

contains the compartments called *cotyledons*.

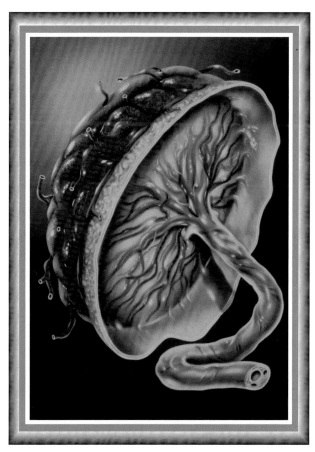

Photo: © John Bavosi / Photo Researchers, Inc. 2006

RHOGAM, FOR Rh NEGATIVE MOMS

As we mentioned earlier, mother's blood and baby's blood do not ever mix. If they did there would be a good chance that the mother would develop a reaction and make *antibodies* that would attack the fetus's blood supply. This is known as *Rh disease*. It occurs when a woman is Rh negative and her husband is Rh positive. If the baby is also Rh positive any mixing of the mother's blood with the baby's will cause her to develop antibodies that will attack the unborn baby's red blood cells. This can cause the baby to be severely *anemic* and require transfusion. In order to prevent this, a mother who is Rh negative is given a *Rhogam* injection just prior to birth or at any time there is a possibility of blood mixing, such as during an amniocentesis. Your healthcare provider will determine your blood type very early during your pregnancy and, if you are Rh negative, will plan your Rhogam injections.

"My mother had a slender, small body, but a large heart — a heart so large that everybody's joys found welcome in it, and hospitable accommodation."

– Mark Twain

MORE HORMONES

As you know by now, hormones play a huge role in your pregnancy. Your *cholesterol*, which is now at a very high level, circulates in the blood as a substance known as *lipoprotein*. The placenta has special receptors for this substance. In this way, cholesterol serves as "raw material" for production by the placenta of massive amounts of hormones.

One of the hormones which influences changes in your breasts and causes relaxation of your uterus and other smooth muscles is *progesterone*. In addition, progesterone is transferred to the fetus who uses it as a building block to make other hormones, particularly the stress hormone *cortisol* and the male hormone *testosterone*.

BABY'S FIRST MEAL

The adrenal glands of the fetus are very important. Adrenal glands sit on top of the kidneys. By late pregnancy, they have each reached the size equivalent to those of an adolescent. After birth, your baby's adrenal glands will shrink dramatically. The fetal adrenal gland makes a male hormone called *androgen* which circulates to the placenta and is changed to a female hormone, *estrogen*. The placenta cannot make large amounts of estrogen without this fetal building-block. Large amounts of estrogen (predominantly an estrogen called *estriol*) in turn, cause the mother to make a breast-stimulating hormone called *prolactin*. In this way the fetus indirectly guarantees itself a meal after birth! Ninety percent of all *estriol* is ultimately derived from this fetal precursor.

Towards the end of this trimester a sticky, watery, milk-like substance known as *colostrum* will be present in your breasts and can usually be expressed from them by hand. This substance will be the baby's first food, since it precedes the arrival of your actual milk supply which usually comes in at two to three days after delivery.

> "Of all the rights of women, the greatest is to be a mother."
>
> – Lin Yutang

NEARING COMPLETION

At the beginning of this trimester your unborn child will be about 10 inches in length (crown-rump height) and weigh about 2 pounds, 12 ounces. It's foot will measures about 2.1 inches, about the size of a large paper clip. His/Her skin will be red and completely covered by *vernix*. Baby fat continues to accumulate beneath the fetus's skin, and the buds of permanent teeth will appear. During this trimester if your baby is male, the testes will descend first to the groin and later into the scrotum. There will be quite a bit of hair present on your baby's head and its eyes will completely open by the end of this trimester. The whole purpose of this trimester is for your baby to keep adding fat and filling out.

"A grandmother is a mother who has a second chance."

– Author Unknown

Calcium levels in the blood of the fetus are actually higher than those in the mother's blood. The placenta has been called a "calcium pump," supplying that mineral from the mother to the fetus who needs great amounts of it in order to form bones. That's why it is so important to maintain good dietary intake of milk, cheese, yogurt and your prenatal vitamins.

Your unborn child is maturing at a rapid rate. While still in the uterus, a fetus of this age has been reported to both vomit and have diarrhea. *After rupture of the bag of waters and introduction of air into the uterus, actual crying of the fetus has been heard!*

By the end of this trimester you unborn child will be about *14½ inches long* (sitting height) and weigh slightly more than *7 pounds*. Its head diameter is expected to be about 9.5 centimeters. His/Her fingernails will reach the fingertips, but toenails do not reach toe tips. The skin will be pink rather than red, and the vernix will be very thick.

THE CORD

The *umbilical cord* measures ½ inch in diameter and 20 inches in length. Inside the cord are two arteries and one vein. The cord resembles a necklace with many spiral twists and in about one-third of babies is wrapped around the baby's neck. This condition is rarely dangerous but can cause the baby's heart rate to slow necessitating a possible cesarean section.

BIRTHMARKS

Birthmarks are a bit of a misnomer because they have nothing to do with the mechanical process of birth, nor are they the result of any trauma. Except in rare instances, a birthmark is not a tumor and will only grow at approximately the same rate as the tissue surrounding it. Some birthmarks persist throughout life, and some regress significantly or disappear entirely during childhood. Any part of the skin may be involved, but over half are found on the face, scalp or neck. New laser equipment has proven successful in removing many such birthmarks.

"To describe my mother would be to write about a hurricane in its perfect power."

– Maya Angelou

This is a full-term infant in the womb.

He will be born with the waxy covering that you see on his head (vernix).

The cord will be clamped and cut and only a small remnant will be left behind.

This remnant will fall off within about 10 days.

It looks like this baby is going to have a full head of hair too.

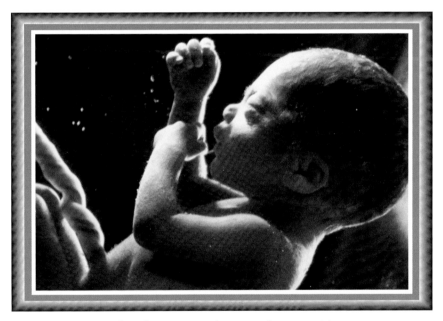

Photo: © Petit Format / Photo Researchers, Inc. 2006

MAKING THINGS EASIER

As the due date approaches, many women have questions for their physicians regarding the mechanics of the birth and medication. While the goal of many women today is an unmedicated or "natural birth," medication can be beneficial to the mother and not harmful to the fetus. Pain relief may sufficiently change a mother's breathing pattern so that the acid content of her blood is better for her baby.

Today, almost one-third of *anesthesia* is related to childbirth. General anesthesia in which the mother inhales a substance to render her unconscious is seldom used for vaginal births, although it is used for emergent cesarean sections when adequate *analgesia* is not obtained through an epidural or there is not time enough to start an epidural anesthetic. A *cesarean*, or C-section, is surgery which accomplishes delivery through the abdomen; about one in seven babies is delivered in this manner.

Regional anesthetics, such as *epidurals* and *spinals* are administered in the spinal or epidural space surrounding the spinal cord. These anesthetics have the advantage of blocking sensation in the lower half of the body but the mother remains awake and alert to assist in the birth and witness it. Epidurals have become very commonplace and most *anesthesiologists* and *nurse anesthetists* are quite expert at placing them.

"A hundred years from now, it will not matter what my bank-account was, the sort of house I lived in, or the make of car I drove. But the world may be different, because I was important in the life of a child."

– Author Unknown

ROOMS WITH A VIEW

While a majority of births still take place in hospitals, there are a growing number of options for delivery. Midwifery is legal and practiced in all 50 states. A *midwife* is a specially trained and licensed nurse who can assist a woman at birth either in a labor and delivery room or if a woman so desires, at home.

Within hospitals, more and more are setting aside special birthing rooms which are furnished much like the bedroom in a private room. Here a woman can labor and deliver in the same bed, with her husband and other family members or siblings present. However, such rooms can only be used by women whose labor is progressing normally with no contraindications such as a rise in maternal blood pressure or the fetus being in an unusual position. Whether giving birth in a traditional labor room or one of the new birthing rooms, most hospitals today welcome husbands or a woman's labor coach. In fact, many hospitals even allow husbands into the operating room if a cesarean section is necessary.

> "Pride is one of the seven deadly sins; but it cannot be the pride of a mother in her children, for that is a compound of two cardinal virtues — faith and hope."
>
> – Charles Dickens in Nicholas Nickleby

HAPPY BIRTHDAY!

Hospitals and the entire medical profession recognize the need to make the birth as private and family-oriented as possible. Regardless of the medical or physical circumstances of your child's birth, it is bound to be one of the most thrilling and joyous experiences of your life – one birthday you'll never forget!

"God sends children for another purpose than merely to keep up the race –

To enlarge our hearts; and to make us unselfish and full of kindly sympathies

and affections; to give our souls higher aims; and to bring round our firesides bright

faces, happy smiles, and loving tender hearts. My soul blesses the great Father every

day, that he has gladdened the earth with little children."

– Mary Howitt 1799 – 1888, English Poet

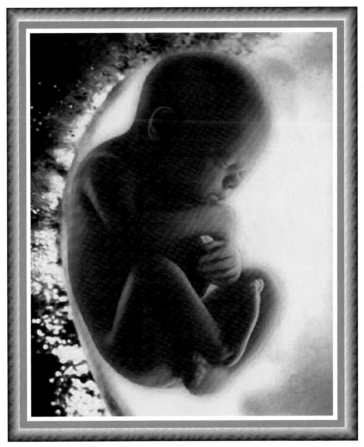

Photo: © Yoav Levy/Phototake 2006

THE AUTHORS

Jack H. McCubbin, MD has delivered thousands of babies and is the author of *The Unborn Baby Book* (published in seven countries) and *The Labor Room Book.* He has written numerous scientific articles and textbook chapters, and has served on the faculty of The University of Texas (Southwestern) Health Science Center, The University of Tennessee College of Medicine, and the University of Arkansas College of Medicine. Dr. McCubbin is a Diplomat of the American Board of Obstetrics and Gynecology, a Fellow of the American College of Obstetricians and Gynecologists, and a Fellow of the American College of Surgeons. He maintains a private practice in Texarkana, Texas, where he lives with his wife, Liza.

Catherine M. Schaffer, PA-C has served as a Clinical Associate with Baylor College of Medicine in the Department of Obstetrics and the Department of Surgery. She has worked extensively with women suffering from high-risk medical problems during pregnancy, as well as women with HIV and substance abuse issues. Ms. Schaffer is the author of many articles on pregnancy, focusing on getting high-risk patients to seek prenatal care. She resides in Bridgeport, New York with her husband, Rich, where she devotes her time to writing and consulting.

INDEX